SpringerBriefs in Food, Health, and Nutrition

Springer Briefs in Food, Health, and Nutrition present concise summaries of cutting edge research and practical applications across a wide range of topics related to the field of food science, including its impact and relationship to health and nutrition. Subjects include:

- Food chemistry, including analytical methods; ingredient functionality; physic-chemical aspects; thermodynamics
- Food microbiology, including food safety; fermentation; foodborne pathogens; detection methods
- Food process engineering, including unit operations; mass transfer; heating, chilling and freezing; thermal and non-thermal processing, new technologies
- Food physics, including material science; rheology, chewing/mastication
- Food policy
- And applications to:
  - Sensory science
  - Packaging
  - Food quality
  - Product development

We are especially interested in how these areas impact or are related to health and nutrition.

Featuring compact volumes of 50 to 125 pages, the series covers a range of content from professional to academic. Typical topics might include:

- A timely report of state-of-the art analytical techniques
- A bridge between new research results, as published in journal articles, and a contextual literature review
- A snapshot of a hot or emerging topic
- An in-depth case study
- A presentation of core concepts that students must understand in order to make independent contributions

For further volumes:
http://www.springer.com/series/10203

Roselina Karim • Muhammad Tauseef Sultan

Yellow Alkaline Noodles

Processing Technology and Quality Improvement

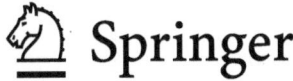 Springer

Roselina Karim
Department of Food Technology, Faculty
of Food Science and Technology,
Universiti Putra Malaysia
Serdang, Selangor
Malaysia

Muhammad Tauseef Sultan
Department of Food Technology, Faculty
of Food Science and Technology,
Universiti Putra Malaysia
Serdang, Selangor
Malaysia

ISSN 2197-571X   ISSN 2197-5728 (electronic)
SpringerBriefs in Food, Health, and Nutrition
ISBN 978-3-319-12864-1   ISBN 978-3-319-12865-8 (eBook)
DOI 10.1007/978-3-319-12865-8

Springer Cham Heidelberg New York Dordrecht London

Printed on acid-free paper

Springer is part of Springer Science+Business Media (www.springer.com)

Preface

Noodles are amongst the oldest forms of processed food consumed and are considered to be important component of human diets especially for the communities living in South East Asia e.g. China, Japan, Indonesia, Malaysia, Thailand, etc. In recent years, noodles have also become popular in other parts of the world and their consumption is increasing with each passing day in some developing economies. The noodles are of various types and wide range of differences exists between communities living in different countries. In general, we can classify them based on origin i.e. Chinese, Japanese, and Thai bamee. They can also be categorized into white and yellow noodles based on their color. Similarly, they can also be classified based on flour type e.g. wheat and rice noodles. The variations in processing techniques also results in sub-classification of noodles into four types i.e. fresh, semi-boiled, dried, boiled, and steamed noodles. Amongst these all types, yellow alkaline noodles are of considerable importance owing to their brightness and yellow color tone. They are famous in South East Asia and now taking share in other parts of the globe too. Noodles and pasta are related products and both of them can be served in the same way. According to the best of authors knowledge, the literature regarding yellow alkaline noodles has not been compiled in the form of book/brief and knowledge is disintegrated that needs to be combined together to bring maximum information at one point. This Springer-brief is an attempt to clarify several issues related to yellow alkaline noodles e.g. classification, ingredients and their role, processing technology, factors affecting the quality of noodles, improving nutritional values, and indeed discussing the modern concepts and innovations. The noodles are of many types and sometime pasta and other products are also placed in the same category. However, there are some differences too that are highlighted in the first proposed heading of this Springer-brief i.e. Introduction and background. A detailed discussion (second heading) regarding noodle classification based on various characteristics is limelight of this Springer-brief. **In the third heading of the proposed brief**, the authors briefed the readers about the yellow alkaline noodles. **In the fourth heading**, the quality criteria have been discussed for each raw material. **In the fifth heading**, the detailed manufacturing has been discussed. **In the 6th & 7th headings**, the discussion has been made regarding the factors affecting the quality of the yellow alkaline noodles along with measure to improve the nutritional value and quality. **In the last heading**, discussion has been made with reference to the modern trends and innovations to brief the readers about the recent developments and future prospects with special reference to preservation. The authors has also mention future prospects and areas of research, thus stakeholders could divert their attention to solve those problems. As we mentioned earlier, there is no book/ brief available on this topic thus there is need to present all the details in comprehensive and lucid manner in one Springer-brief. I hope that the present springer brief would be interesting for the readers and allied stakeholders.

Dr. Roselina Karim

Contents

Contents

Chapter 1
Background and Introduction

Noodles are one of the oldest forms of processed food consumed and it constitutes an important component of diets of communities living in South East Asia, for example, China, Japan, Indonesia, Malaysia, and Thailand. In recent years, noodles have also become popular and their consumption is increasing with each passing day in other parts of the world, for example developing economies like India and Pakistan. The developed and emerging economies like the USA, Mexico, Brazil, and European countries are promising markets for noodles. As per one global estimate, more than 1 billion meals containing noodles were served in the last year thus showing the rapid growing market (WINA 2013).

Consumers should not be confused between noodles and pasta, as these two terms are used interchangeable over the globe. However, these are two different products, as pasta is usually prepared from durum wheat and noodles are manufactured from common wheat. Pasta is one generic term that includes variety of products including macaroni, spaghetti, ravioli, lasagna, vermicelli, and egg macaroni. Most of the time, pasta and allied products are made up of durum wheat or semolina and water which are passed through a die at higher pressure (extrusion process) after mixing, while noodles are not extruded products. The serving method is also different for both products. Noodles may be served in variety of forms that may include raw, partially boiled, boiled, dried, steamed, and fried. In contrast, pasta is normally distributed in dried forms. Although, some types of noodles like dried noodle matches in some textural characteristics with pasta products but this is not the case with all of the noodles (Cole 1991; Hou 2001).

As mentioned earlier, noodles and allied products are dietary staples for communities living in South East Asia and spreading to whole globe with ~7% annual growth. However, historical background suggests the art of noodle making belongs to Chinese communities. Later, the noodles gained immense popularity in closer vicinities like Japan, Malaysia, Indonesia, Thailand, Burma, and India (Fu 2008; Hou 2010). In the present era, noodles form one of the main dishes in Malaysian diet too and can be served in many forms, and are frequently taken

© The Authors 2015
R. Karim, M. T. Sultan, *Yellow Alkaline Noodles,* SpringerBriefs in Food,
Health, and Nutrition, DOI 10.1007/978-3-319-12865-8_1

as a replacement for rice during the main meals or in between meals. Overall, noodles are very popular among all races especially the Malaysian Chinese. The amount of noodles consumed is large and it contributes around 30% of total flour used in Malaysia (Hou 2010). Noodles also occupy an important place in the people living in the USA. According to an estimate, annual per capita noodle consumption has been reported at 304.1 g/day. Moreover, the annual consumption of noodles has jumped to 101,420 million bags/cups annually (Chung et al. 2010; WINA 2013).

The noodles and related pasta products industry forms one of the major food manufacturing industries in Malaysia. Almost all of the factories produced noodles for local consumption. Most of the processing plants operate on small scale and some of them performed in the backyard. The production of these products mostly involved batch processing operations but in some cases modern continues automated processing plants are installed. The number of establishments involved in the manufacture of noodles and related pasta products in Peninsular Malaysia increased from 245 to 396 with gross value output of $ 30,198 and $ 116,003 respectively. The upward tendency reflects the bright future ahead. There is a considerable variation in the quality of noodles produce in this country, depending upon the manufacturer, techniques used and the consumer demands. Preferences for color, texture, and taste vary with different ethnic groups and method of serving. Manufacturers are often required to produce different characteristics of noodles as a result of consumer demand. In Malaysia, different types of noodles and pasta are available in the market and they are manufactured using the wheat/rice flour (Hou 2010).

The yellow alkaline noodles are popular form of food that is responsible for 48% of flour consumption in South East Asia. It is essentially stripe cut from of a sheet of dough that comprised of wheat flour, water, common salt, and alkaline salts. Some optional ingredients like eggs, milk, and meat are also utilized to give specific taste and aroma depending upon the demands of the consumers. During noodle making process, the dough is pressed between combining rollers and sheeted several times before being cut into strips. They are having pH in the range of 9–11 thus having limited shelf life (~2–3 days under refrigerated storage). Sometimes, eggs are added depending upon the type of noodles being made. The utilization of natural preservatives are also gaining wide range of application in such noodles (Chang and Wu 2008; Rosyid et al. 2011). These noodles are usually shaped into slender strips with array of variations in their size and length (Hatcher et al. 2009a; Gulia et al. 2014).

The widespread consumptions of noodles have led to significant developments across the world that is not only confined to the noodle industry but also important for wheat breeder and producers, thus they can develop such wheat cultivars which can meet the requirements of the noodles industry. Similarly, the milling industries are also responding with better quality of the wheat flour. Moreover, the engineering companies dealing in equipments and processing tools are also modifying the processing in order to maximize the returns for all stakeholders (Konik et al. 1994; Okusu et al. 2010; Park et al. 2011).

According to the best of authors knowledge, the literature regarding yellow alkaline noodles has not been compiled in the form of book/brief and knowledge is dispersed that needs to be combined together to bring maximum information at one point. This Springer-brief is an attempt to clarify several issues related to yellow alkaline noodles, for example, classification, ingredients and their role, processing technology, factors affecting the quality of noodles, improving nutritional values, and indeed discussing the modern concepts and innovations.

Chapter 2
Types of Noodles: A Brief Description

As mentioned earlier that noodles are becoming an important component of human diet. However, they are served in different forms and shapes depending upon the preferences of the communities. Moreover, there are several variations with special reference to the ingredients, processing techniques, and end use quality. The noodles are of many types and sometime pasta and other products are also placed in the same category of cereal products. Although, some discussion has been made in the introduction section to highlight the differences between noodles and pasta but differences among different noodles need further elaborations. For the purpose, a brief and concise discussion regarding noodle classification based on various characteristics has been made in this heading.

Since ancient times, there many types of noodles available in the market and different regions thus making the classification more complicated. Generally, noodles are classified into various types and there exists wide range of differences among different communities living in different countries. In general, we can classify them based on origin, that is, Chinese, Japanese, Korean, Italian, and Thai bamee noodles. They can be categorized into white and yellow noodles based on their color. Similarly, they can also be classified based on flour type, for example, wheat and rice noodles. The instant noodles have become an important component of global diet. The variations in processing techniques also results in subclassification of noodles into four types, that is, fresh, dried, boiled, and steamed noodles. Commonly utilized noodles in Malaysia include yellow alkaline noodles sold (boiled/semiboiled) in different forms, that is, Cantonese and Hokkein noodles. Apart from these noodles, other types of noodles that are commonly consumed by Malaysian and other peoples in South East Asia are starch vermicelli, kuay teow, rice noodles, and Korean style noodles. The noodles like lo shee fund, chee cheon fun, kuay teow are also important (Fu 2008; Okusu et al. 2010; Heo et al. 2012; Gulia et al. 2014). Similar to the classification, nomenclature differs accordingly. In China, wheat is usually called as mein and rice as fun thus noodles with wheat as main ingredient are called as mein and rice noodles are called as fun. Noodles prepared with starch extracted from different sources are labeled as vermicelli (Galvez and Ressurreccion 1992).

© The Authors 2015
R. Karim, M. T. Sultan, *Yellow Alkaline Noodles,* SpringerBriefs in Food,
Health, and Nutrition, DOI 10.1007/978-3-319-12865-8_2

Among, yellow alkaline noodles are prepared from wheat flour along with water and alkaline salt as their basic ingredients. However, there are some differences with special reference to the Chinese noodles as they are boiled partially. In this regard, noodles prepared with the addition of egg (wantan noodles) are also popular which are parboiled using steam and dried. The noodles are divided into two major categories, that is, white or Japanese noodle, and yellow or Chinese noodles. Japanese noodles are made from flour of weak strength that may contain around 9.0–11.0 % of proteins contents. They also include the salts and water. They are white colored thicker noodles as compared to yellow colored thin Chinese noodles. These both are sold dried or boiled form, however, yellow alkaline noodles are usually sold in wet form containing moisture contents in the range of 50–60 % (final product). Chinese noodles are made from wheat flour that should contain protein contents in the range of 10–13 % but preferable protein contents are in the range 11–12 % (Zhao and Seib 2005). These noodles also include alkaline lye that is also called as kansui (mixture of sodium/potassium carbonate and bicarbonate), common salt, and water. Cantonese, Hokkein, and wantan noodles are some forms of yellow alkaline noodles available in the market. Cantonese styled noodles are one category which act as a basic ingredient for the preparation of others noodles. These noodles are sold uncooked or raw and if they are dried, they are known as dried noodles. Hokkein styled noodles are raw Chinese noodles which have been boiled for few minutes (parboiled) until there is only fine core of dough in the center surrounded by cooked or gelatinized dough. They are also known as partially boiled noodles or wet noodles. Wantan style noodles are Chinese noodles in which eggs are incorporated as one of the major ingredient. They are also sold with brand name of egg noodles and sold in wet forms. Finally, instant noodles are raw noodles which are steamed for few minutes and then dried in the sun or heating cabinet (Hou 2010).

Chapter 3
Yellow Alkaline Noodles: An Introduction

Yellow alkaline noodles are of considerable importance owing to their brightness and yellow color tone. Generally, yellow alkaline noodles are commonly consumed in South East Asia (Indonesia, Malaysia, Singapore, Thailand, etc.) and Japan. They are made from wheat flour, water, salt and alkaline salt, and are usually parboiled. The presence of alkaline salt contributes to the yellow color, firm texture, alkaline flavor, and high pH to the noodles. There are again many forms of alkaline noodles and the most popular forms are fresh, dried, wet/boiled, and noodles with egg added as ingredient. They vary mainly in the method of manufacturing especially at the final stages/steps. Wet yellow alkaline (Hokkien) noodles are popular in Malaysia, Indonesia, Singapore, and can be found in Asian market. Hokkien noodles generally have a moisture content of 50–60 %. The presence of higher moisture contents is significant feature of these types of noodles that also limit their shelf life to $1-1.5$ days. However, the proper processing and packaging can enhance the shelf life of the noodles up to 3–4 days (Fu 2008; Gulia et al. 2014).

Textural profile of the noodles varies greatly but smoothness, firmness, stickiness, cohesiveness, elasticity, chewiness, and gumminess are among the important parameters (Deng et al. 2008; Hatcher et al. 2009b). The instrumental techniques to measure textural profile include simple compression testing and texture profile analyzer (TPA). The details regarding textural profile are mentioned in subsequent headings.

The major hindrance regarding the growth of yellow alkaline noodles is their shelf life. Although, it can be increased to 3–4 days under refrigerated storage and proper packaging but quality tends to decrease during storage. In general, the quality of raw material is important especially wheat flour that should contain ~ 12 % gluten protein. Mostly, the common alkaline salt used is sodium carbonate but mixtures of sodium and potassium carbonate are most common in Japan. The amount and type of alkaline salts are of significant importance as they impart yellowish tonality and slight brightness. The amount of kansui added is normally 1 %, but can be increased up to 1.5 % based on the weight of flour (Morris et al. 2000). The amount of other

© The Authors 2015
R. Karim, M. T. Sultan, *Yellow Alkaline Noodles,* SpringerBriefs in Food,
Health, and Nutrition, DOI 10.1007/978-3-319-12865-8_3

ingredients added is normally 1–2 % depending on the weight of flour and consumer preferences. The amount of water remains in the range of 28–35 % of flour weight (Zhao and Seib 2005; Gulia et al. 2014). Generally, some significant features of alkaline noodles include bright and appealing yellow color with exceptional flavor and textural profile (Zhao and Seib 2005).

Chapter 4
Raw Materials and Their Quality

Noodles are usually manufactured using different raw materials, such as rice, mung-bean, sweet potato, potato starch, tapioca, sago, buckwheat, and wheat. The most popular noodles among Asian peoples are the one, which uses wheat flour as the main ingredient. According to one estimate, around 40 % of the flour consumed in Asia is used to make noodles. The ingredients like common salt, alkaline salt, and water also play an important role in end use quality.

4.1 Wheat Flour

Wheat is primary and foremost important component of noodles. The quality of wheat is dependent on its type, genetic makeup and environmental variables. The wheat can be classified into three genotypes that is diploid (having two set of chromosomes), tetraploid (having four set of chromosomes), and hexaploid (having six set of chromosomes). The common wheat is hexaploid and durum wheat is tetraploid in nature. The common wheat (*Triticum aestivum*) is further divided into various types, that is soft and hard wheat, based on hardness. Wheat can be classified on the basis of color, season of cultivation, etc. However, classification into soft and hard wheat is usually more preferred due to their distinct utilizations. In terms of noodle processing, soft wheat is used for the preparation of white salted noodles and hard wheat is used for the preparation of yellow alkaline noodles. In general, wheat grain comprised of three parts (~75–82 % endosperm, ~12–16 % bran, and ~2–3 % germ) having different chemical composition, thus affecting the products. The endosperm usually harbor storage proteins and starch granules and these two play important roles in flour and end product quality. The branny portion comprise of enzymatic protein, minerals, vitamins, nonstarch polysaccharides, etc. In contrast to these two, wheat germ contains appreciable quantity of good quality protein, edible oils/fats, and vitamins. Among these, endosperm is more important for the

© The Authors 2015
R. Karim, M. T. Sultan, *Yellow Alkaline Noodles*, SpringerBriefs in Food,
Health, and Nutrition, DOI 10.1007/978-3-319-12865-8_4

Table 4.1 Quality parameters of wheat and wheat flour

Sr. no.	Types of parameters	Examples
1	Grain quality parameters	Grain size, grain hardness, grain weight, grain shape and test weight
2	Physical parameters	Flour yield, pearling value, sizing produced, purity, sedimentation test
3	Chemical parameters	Wheat proteins, moisture, fats, carbohydrates, gluten, high molecular gluten proteins, falling number
4	Rheological parameters	Farinographic characters (mixing tolerance index, water absorption, dough development time, dough stability time), mixographic characters (mixing time, mixing tolerance index)

production of wheat flour suitable for noodles and allied products. Its amount is also an indicator of flour yield, as higher the endosperm results in higher yield and vice versa (Wang et al. 2008; Shewry 2009).

The wheat grading systems are also important in determining the milling and end use quality of wheat products. There are several parameters used for the grading that may include thousand grain weight, damaged grains, broken grains, presence of foreign material, grains from other cereals, insect damage & excreta, etc. However, these parameters are used for grading of wheat and they cannot be termed as criteria for evaluating the flour quality. The quality assessment of wheat flour that is again dependent on wheat includes several quality parameters. A brief description has been presented as under. (Table 4.1)

These parameters can be of physical/chemical nature, that is, moisture, protein, ash, fiber, gluten, and starch contents. In this regard, Ahmad et al. (2007) and Arif et al. (2006) evaluated wheat varieties of Pakistan and observed that these cultivars differ significantly from each other, for example, protein content varied from 10.0 to 14.8 % (Arif et al. 2006; Zeb et al. 2006; Ahmad et al. 2007). The starch pasting properties, amylose/amylopectin ratio, farinographic characteristics, and damaged starch are also of considerable importance (Hatcher et al. 2002).

As far as measurement of wheat quality is concerned, various instruments are available at different research centers and laboratories. The test includes sodium dodecyl sulphate (SDS) sedimentation test, dry and wet gluten, viscosity, specific absorbance, starch pasting characteristics, rheological characteristics, etc. The principle factors that governed the eating quality of noodles are protein content, starch characteristics, dough strength, and paste viscosity (Huang and Morrison 1988; Huang and Lai 2010; Ross and Crosbie 2010).

The researchers across the globe concluded that protein quantity and quality are prerequisite for superior cooking quality (Park et al. 2003). A positive correlation can be observed for SDS sedimentation and noodle quality and negative proportionality with alcohol and salt soluble wheat proteins (Park and Baik 2004). The color of noodles besides being affected by the presence of both brown and yellow pigments and the branny specks in flour is also influenced by the protein content of flours

(Jiang et al. 2011). The most of technological properties related to dough making and baking are dependent upon the wheat proteins. Protein contents of wheat flour are dependent on genetic classification, environmental factors, extraction rate, etc. However, flour used for yellow alkaline noodles usually contains 11.0–13.5 % proteins (Zhao and Seib 2005; Ye et al. 2009). The gluten proteins constitute ~ 80 % of proteins present in wheat flour. They are further comprised of two districts types, that is, gliadin and glutenin. The gliadin fractions are important in formation of disulfide bonds thus rendering firmness against aggregate formation, while glutenin are elastic in nature. These two proteins combine together to form gluten network. Gliadin fraction forms disulfide linkages and glutenin fraction give elasticity and extensibility to the dough. The higher amount of glutenin enhances the viscoelastic properties of wheat flour, while higher amounts of gliadin are negative correlated with the said trait. However, the chemistry of such proteins are not as simple and glutenin proteins are further categorized into low molecular weight glutenin (LMW) proteins and high molecular weight glutenin (HMW) proteins. Both these subtypes possess distinct properties for different cereal products but HMW composition is more important for bread making and end use quality of wheat flour. Although, HMW glutenin is present in lower quantities but plays an important role during mixing thus mixing time, dough stability, and dough development time are positively correlated with such fractions (Veraverbeke and Delcour 2002; Yamauchi et al. 2007; Ong et al. 2010).

Starch is a major constituent of wheat flour contributing to about 75 % of the total composition. It can be considered an important source of dietary energy of the noodles, usually contributing around 70 % of total energy obtained from such yellow alkaline noodles. Starch plays various roles in the food products including bulking, thickener, stabilizer, texture modifier, etc. The starch granules present in wheat flour usually varies from 8 to 20 μm in size. The starch, as many readers know comprised of two distinct side chains, that is, amylose and amylopectin. These chains differ in their molecular chemistry and degree of polymerization. The starch granules contain some minor amounts of phosphates too that impart some significant functional properties. The amylose and amylopectin differs significantly in their functional properties. Amylose form stable and firmer gel that sets quite early. In contrast, amylopectin form stable but clear viscous gels. Amylose retrogrades easily but amylopectin is quite stable. Some of starch sources like mung beans and sago contain more amounts of amylopectin thus, their swelling properties and stability during mixing and other processes make them suitable for the preparation of starch noodles. The swelling power test can also be used to select the suitable varieties for yellow alkaline noodles (Toyokawa et al. 1989b; McCormick et al. 1991; Rayas-Duarte et al. 2009).

Starches with lower amylose contents are more suitable for the production of noodles. Generally, the starch provides a platform for its attachment with gluten strand. In simplistic language, it can be claimed that gluten form the basic dough by forming a strong bond with added water. Later, the starch swells and gelatinizes after heating thus, working as building block for final baked product. During mixing and dough development, gluten retains maximum of absorbed water. Later, the starch helps in maintaining the final shape of products by setting the gluten structure, that is, making it rigid by drawing away water especially from gluten during gelatinization. It can be termed that the starch granules act as filler in the dough system thus, providing gluten as the desirable consistency (Akashi et al. 1999; Baik and Lee 2003).

The interactions between different components like proteins, starch, enzymes, nonstarch polysaccharides, etc. are important for determining the quality of end product (Toyokawa et al. 1989a). The flour quality is also linked with the eating quality of the noodles too. Although, the exact relationship between the flour characteristics and eating quality is yet to be determined but still many researchers have presented evidences and some parameters are positively correlated with the eating qualities of the noodles.

4.2 Water

Water is an essential ingredient necessary for gluten formation which provides viscoelastic properties to dough required for noodle processing. Water is the ingredient most responsible for the biochemical and physical interaction that occurs in foods. Yet, many of us tend to underestimate or overlook its importance. The gluten network formation based on water hydration is not as consistent in noodle dough as in bread dough. The water contents of noodles dough ranging from 28 to 35 % allow formation of a continuous gluten matrix, rendering them less susceptible to gluten breakdown. The scientists confirmed this hypothesis after analyzing the dough using scanning electron microscopy. The formation of continuous network of protein sheets and fibrils did not occur in yellow alkaline noodles dough to the same extent as in the bread dough (Park and Baik 2002). The water absorption level recommended for noodle processing is about 28–35 % based on flour weight. During processing, water level can be used to control the dough strength and thereby, significantly influence machineability in products requiring molding and to assure proper texture of the final product (Hatcher et al. 1999). In commercial manufacturing of noodles, the level of water used depends on the various ingredients in the formula, processing equipment, processing variable, and on the characteristics required in the noodle product. In predicting the optimum water absorption of flour, several testing procedures are used and amongst water absorption determined through Farinograph is important. If water is added in less amounts than the recommended levels, the harder and stiffer dough will form that can withstand the pressure during subsequent pressure of sheeting and molding. The insufficient water levels also results in nonuniform white patches of flour on the surface of yellow alkaline noodles. In contrast to lower levels, amount of water added in higher amounts than the recommended results in dough of low viscosity and higher stickiness. The sticky dough creates problems during subsequent operations like sheeting and cutting. Moreover, the noodles strips stretches more thus enhancing the cooking losses (Huang and Lai 2010).

The presence of impurities and salts results in water hardness that can also influence the end product quality. Water hardness is linked with the presence of calcium, sulphates, magnesium cations, bicarbonates, etc. However, the scientists didn't provide enough information to study the effects of harness on the physicochemical and chemical features of noodles. Hardness of water has been shown to influence the cooking quality of noodles and noodles cooked in deionized water had a better firmer surface than those cooked in tap water. Calcium and magnesium at pH 9.2 and at the concentration found in tap water had little effect on surface firmness and cooking loss. However, higher levels of calcium and magnesium can increase the surface firmness of cooked noodles. Quality of cooking water has large influence on stickiness of cooked spaghetti. Cooking water hardness increased the stickiness of spaghetti and vice versa. Moreover, the cooking loss tended to increase accordingly. Moreover, the alkalinity and water hardness solubilized the starch to a greater extend thus giving rise to higher cooking losses. The cooking loss is in direct proportionality with the pH of the water, for example, pH toward alkalinity results in higher water loss. The increase in cooking loss is due to swelling of gluten which results in weak association with starch thus, the surface firmness decreases thus opening the matrix that contributes to the cooking loss. Noodles become very sticky when the pH of water increased to 9.0–9.5. Size and general appearance of the noodles are not influenced by the increase in pH of the precooking water. However, the overall cross section of partly cooked noodles increased with alkali buildup. From these studies, it appears that alkalinity of cooking water affected the periphery of the noodle structure. The addition of wheat and processing conditions, the pH of cooking water is also responsible for the changes in eating quality of noodles. Alkalinity of cooking water was observed to exert its effect more on stickiness and surface disintegration. The alkalinity has more effects on pasta and related products as compared to yellow alkaline noodles. In yellow alkaline noodles, the pH is always around 9.0–11.0 and consumer preferences are also align accordingly.

4.3 Alkaline Salts

One of the most essential ingredients in yellow alkaline noodles preparation beside flour, water, and sodium chloride is alkaline lye that is also called "kansui". The alkalizing agents consist of sodium/potassium carbonate or bicarbonate or a mixture of any or all of these salts. The type and proportion of salts in the alkaline lye depends on the manufacturers themselves. In some cases, sodium hydroxide, sodium silicate, or even borax are incorporated. However, borax and allied products are banned in the past few years due to its side effects on human health. The alkaline salts confer a unique flavor and quality to the yellow alkaline noodles. These salts react with the phytochemicals especially the flavones of wheat starch thus develop yellow color. In the noodle manufacturing process, the alkaline salts increase the toughness of dough. The alkali resulted in noodles that were brighter and much yellower than the noodles form salted dough (Morris et al. 2000). Alkaline dough developed and broke down more rapidly in the farinograph, and tougher and less extensible in the extensorgraph test (Zhang et al. 2011).

In this regard, various scientists studied the role of alkaline salts and their impact on noodles quality. In one such study, Shelke et al. (1990) estimated the effects of different amounts of alkaline salts and their impact on quality of wet noodles. Later, Kruger et al. (1992) determined the association of alkaline salts and yellow color of alkaline noodles. The yellow alkaline noodles using 1 % sodium hydroxide were the brightest and yellowest but they resulted in the formation of softer and slightly sticky dough. Actually, sodium hydroxide also affected the gluten activity as it acted as surfactant thus reducing the surface tension of the water, resulting in less developed dough. However, the starch granules swelled to the greater extent and thus disturbing the protein network. The cooked noodles containing other alkaline salt such combinations of sodium carbonate and potassium carbonate were firmer and more elastic than those made with sodium chloride and sodium hydroxide. Internal firmness and cutting stress of cooked dry noodles can also be affected primarily by the pH of dough. The increase in internal strength of noodles at alkaline pH agreed with the strengthening of wheat dough at alkaline pH. Alkaline conditions in the preparation of noodles modify the properties of dough. It accelerate the process of gelatinization and increase the viscosity of starch paste and hence, affect the color and cooking quality as well as the texture and surface of the final product (Hung and Hatcher 2011).

4.4   Sodium Chloride

Sodium chloride addition is important to impact specific taste and addition of salt in noodle dough includes the tightening of gluten structure, improving the viscoelastic properties, and increasing the water permeability during cooking. It also helps in preventing cracking during drying, suppressing of lactic acid and alcoholic fermentation, and imparting astringency. It exerts its effects on gluten proteins by decreasing the solubility of gluten and results in compaction and exclusions of nonpolar lipids from the hydrophobic interior of the gluten. In this regard, Morris et al. (2002) optimize the formulations of yellow alkaline noodles and recommended 2 % for optimum quality. Later, Hatcher and Anderson (2007) reported the negative effects of sodium chloride when used in quantities higher than 3.0 %. Later, Ye et al. (2009) also studied the effects of salts on yellow alkaline noodles. According to them, the salt can be added from 0 to 2 % but optimum flavor quality can only be achieved at 1.0 % concentration. Overall, it can be concluded that the addition of salt in higher amounts (>2.0 %) effect dough characteristics negatively thus causing deteriorations in dough properties.

The concentration of salt can affect the rheological properties of the dough. However, such effects are dependent on pH, for example at lower pH, there can be remarkable drop in extensibility of dough. The addition of salts tends to increase the hydrophilic interactions and dispersion of the particles in water. The increase in hydrophilic properties could result from disruption of complex involving polyvalent metal ions, particular complex lipids. The presence of salts in the dough of Japanese noodles resulted in soft and sloppy due to sprouted damage wheat flour was improved the quality.

4.5 Functional Ingredients

A bright and light yellow color is desirable for yellow alkaline noodles. Processing factors like steaming, frying or drying, and oil absorption affect the color and flavor of the noodles. Alkaline reagents give a yellowish color tonality to the noodles. The enzymes like transglutaminase can be added in the flour to reduce the process of darkening. Moreover, antimicrobial agents from antura sources can also be added to improve the shelf life along with proving nonnutritive phytochemicals (Rosyid et al. 2011). Flavor is an important parameter governing instant noodle quality. Oil quality is the major determinant of flavor in instant fried noodles as it is responsible for imparting a distinct flavor to noodles. Texture and color assessed using instrumental analysis are important in this regard and are valuable research tools well suited for monitoring noodle quality after changes in formulations, raw materials, and processing (Hatcher et al. 2008a).

Chapter 5
Processing Technology

The processing of noodles looks simple but it requires skills and knowledge to obtain the desired quality with better consumer acceptability. The processing slightly differs at home scale and industrial manufacturing of yellow alkaline noodles. It should be kept in mind that currently yellow alkaline noodles are coming more from cottage industry than multinational and large-scale processing unit. One of the prime reason for this scenario is the lower shelf life of the yellow alkaline noodles. If we look at household level, the basic steps for production of yellow alkaline noodles are weighing of ingredients, dissolving the salts in water, mixing in different speeds, resting, sheeting and compounding, slitting, cooking/parboiling, rinsing and cooling, and oiling. There is little gluten development during the mixing step, since the water level is relatively low, resulting in the formation of crumbly dough with small and uniform particle size. After mixing, the dough is rested for 20–40 min before compounding (Moss et al. 1986). The dough-resting step is required to enable a uniform penetration of water into dough particles, resulting in smoother and less streaky dough as the protein mellows, and becomes more extensible (Morris et al. 2000). The compressed sheet passes through a series of rollers thus reducing the thickness. Later, the specialized cutters further shape the sheet into desirable width with a slitter. In some areas, the process of sheeting and cutting is carried out using the same machine. Wet yellow alkaline noodles are usually parboiled for 60–90 s to achieve 80–90 % gelatinization of starch. Several important steps need to be taken to ensure optimal cooking quality.

The industries with various mechanical and auxiliary facilities are also taking a lion share in the yellow alkaline noodles. The basic steps for production of yellow alkaline noodles are the same as mentioned in the last paragraph, that is mixing, resting, sheeting and compounding, slitting, cooking, rinsing and cooling, and oiling. Mixing of ingredients is often carried out in a horizontal or vertical mixer for 10–15 min (Hou and Kruk 1998). After mixing, the dough is rested for 20–40 min before compounding (Hou and Kruk 1998). Examination of the microstructure of rested dough showed the formation of a more uniform protein matrix with fewer air spaces compared to the normal dough. The dough is then rolled after pressing it

© The Authors 2015
R. Karim, M. T. Sultan, *Yellow Alkaline Noodles*, SpringerBriefs in Food, Health, and Nutrition, DOI 10.1007/978-3-319-12865-8_5

through a pair of rollers for several times to form the noodles sheet. The compressed sheet is reduced stepwise in thickness by passing through a series of rollers which have a gradually reducing gap between them. Roller gap is normally reduced up to 25% for each pass. The partially developed gluten network reaches to full maturity, fully developed during this processing stage. Noodles slitting is done using a cutting roll or a machine which is equipped with a pair of calibration rolls, a slitter, and a cutter or a waver (Hou and Kruk 1998). The final dough thickness is set on the calibration rolls and measured using a thickness dial gauge. The sheet is cut into desirable width with a slitter. Noodles can either be in the form of square or rectangular in shape, depending on the ratio of width to thickness. Noodle strands are usually cut into desirable length by using a cutter. Wet yellow alkaline noodles are usually parboiled for 45–90 s to achieve 80–90% gelatinization of starch. Several important steps need to be taken to ensure optimal cooking quality suggested by Hou and Kruk (1998).

Chapter 6
Factor Affecting Quality of Yellow Alkaline Noodles

In assessing the quality of noodles and past products, various factors such as color, appearance, cooking quality, and physical properties of both the cooked and uncooked products are considered. The selection of quality criteria for any product is dependent upon the preference of the consumers. Likewise, the same quotient is applicable for yellow alkaline noodles (YAN) where raw materials and the preference of the consumers are important to determine its quality. Generally, factors that are associated with the quality characteristics of noodles contribute to the overall acceptance of the consumers. All these factors are equally important and none should be overlooked in any situation. In this regard, the example of Japanese peoples and their preferences for the noodles can clear the reader's concepts. Japanese communities like bright colored noodles with smooth and slippery surfaces instead of hard, rough, or adhering mouth feel. There should be balanced feel of elasticity, stickiness, and softness. The preferences for external characters also include smooth surfaces, bright color, and indeed there should be no bran specks on the surfaces (Jun et al. 1998).

The discussion regarding the factors affecting the quality of YAN is very lengthy. However, it should be kept in mind that it all depends upon the type of the noodle. The quality is dependent on the various factors effects of the raw materials and processing techniques. The quality of noodles generally depends upon the flour characteristics, proportions of ingredients, and conditions used during preparation, or processing variables. There are many factors that affect the quality of YAN including raw materials, processing techniques, environmental factors, and marketing factors. However, the consumer preferences are of considerable importance. Briefly, eating quality, textural properties, cooking quality, and color tonality are important quality determinants. Color is one of the most important quality parameters for noodles because it is the first characteristic perceived by consumers. There are two distinct aspects of color in YAN, that is, brightness and yellowness. Asian consumers prefer bright YAN with less discoloration within 48 h. Yellowness of noodles is usually attributed to the naturally occurring flavones in flour that react with alkaline salts, while the brightness of noodles is due to the flour protein, pigments, or branny specks in flour (Asenstorfer et al. 2006). However, manufacturers might also add

© The Authors 2015
R. Karim, M. T. Sultan, *Yellow Alkaline Noodles,* SpringerBriefs in Food, Health, and Nutrition, DOI 10.1007/978-3-319-12865-8_6

artificial natural colorant to intensify the yellowness of the noodles because natural flour pigmentation is insufficient to meet customer expectations. The most important consideration of the overall noodles' eating quality is textural characteristic, because it determines the overall consumers' acceptability of the product. Asian peoples prefer YAN with firm and elastic texture. Other factors that influence consumers' preference of noodles are the shape and surface appearance. The cooking quality may be defined as the ability to resist disintegration upon prolonged boiling, coupled with a satisfactory degree of cooking and tenderness in the finished product. The other criterion of cooking quality is cooking loss that refers to the amount of solid released from the noodles strands into the cooking water.

Generally, the quality of noodles is dependent on the raw materials used. Among these raw materials wheat flour and its components are foremost important (Bhattacharya and Corke 1996). According to the researchers across, flour with higher dough resistance, higher protein content, lower maltose figure, and adequate starch pasting strength produces YAN with desirable firmness and elasticity (Gulia et al. 2014). The role of protein in flour on the quality characteristics of noodles has been extensively investigated by many researchers across the globe. The amount of proteins especially glaidin and glutenin affects the noodles quality (Deng et al. 2008; Foo et al. 2011). The Japanese noodles require proteins in the amounts of 9.0–11.0%, while YAN require wheat flour which contains proteins in the amounts of 11.0–13.0%. The utilization of alkaline salts result in higher alkaline pH that influence the dough strength thus lower proteins contents in wheat flour results in poor textural characteristics. In contrast, the optimum flour protein content required for making Japanese noodles is 9–11% which is actually the amount just sufficient for the noodle dough to remain intact during manufacture. Protein contents also influence the cooking quality and tolerance to overcooking as they affect the rheological and textural properties. Moreover, the quality and quantity of wheat proteins also play important roles on cooking quality. The addition of some other proteins like egg albumin or glutenin or glaidin also affects the quality of YAN. However, higher protein contents also results in poor color tonality as increasing the proteins beyond 13.0% results in less brightness and yellowish tonality. One of the reason could be the activities of proteolytic enzymes, that is, polyphenol oxidase (PPO). Higher the proteins, higher would be PPO activity. Basically, the PPO originates from bran fraction that might act on tyrosine group in the protein and on other phenolic-type materials occurring naturally in flours to form dark compounds referred as melanin thus reducing the brightness and yellowish color tonality (Zhao and Seib 2005; Fuerst et al. 2006; Asenstorfer et al. 2014). Apart from the protein and starch components, other properties of flour which influence the quality characteristics of noodles are flour granulation and extraction rate. Flour extraction rate did not produce detrimental effect on the textural properties of the noodles. However, extraction rate of flour appears to influence the color of the final product. In this regard, Ye et al. (2009) demonstrated that the extraction rate influence the color and texture of noodles significantly. Moreover, they observed significant improvement for different sensory parameters (appearance, firmness, and smoothness). Moreover, water absorption increased from 33 to 37% at extraction rates of 50 and 70% respectively. However, noodle flavor significantly deteriorated at higher salt concentrations. According to them, the ideal composition for laboratory preparation of Chinese noodles is 60% flour extraction, 35% water addition, and 1% salt concentration.

Water absorption is an important rheological trait that affects the quality of noodles. It has major impact on the mechanical input required for proper processing in order to retain the quality. It is dependent on the ingredients and their functional components, for example, protein and starch of wheat flour. The water absorption affects the textural properties of the dough and noodles (Edwards et al. 1996). It is worthwhile to mention that even water exceeding 2–3% of optimum level is not desirable. It should be kept in mind that the gluten development and its good adhesion with starch granules is prerequisite for optimum noodle quality (Hatcher et al. 2008b). The Brabdender Farinograph is an instrument used to predict the water absorption of wheat flour. The water absorption indicates that presence of damaged starch or nonstarch polysaccharides (Gulia et al. 2014).

Color is one of the most important quality parameters for noodles because it is the first characteristic perceived by consumers. The color of the noodles is dependent upon the raw materials used as illustrated previously. There are two distinct aspects of color in YAN which are brightness and yellowness. Asian consumers prefer bright YAN with less discoloration within 48 h. Yellowness of noodles is usually attributed to the naturally occurring flavones in flour that reacted with kansui, while the brightness of noodles is due to the flour protein, pigments, or branny specks in flour. The higher color pigments in the wheat flour can result in improved color tonality of the noodles (Hou and Kruk 1998). Several instrumental methods are available to screen the color of noodles, that is, Lovibond, Hunterlab, CIElab Space color meter. However, color of the flour can be measured through the Flour Color Grader, Pekar test. Color of YAN is usually measured by spectrocolorimeter (HunterLab colorimeter or CIELab space color meter) in terms of L^* (noodle brightness or lightness), a^* (noodle redness), and b^* (noodle yellowness) color scale. The factors affecting L^* of instant noodles includes the wheat proteins that also exhibit a significant relationship with b^* (Park and Baik 2004). The presence of higher amounts of ash in wheat flour and PPO activity also influences mainly noodle whiteness. The yellowish color of the noodles is attributed to the presence of natural flavonoids pigments, which are colorless at acidic pH levels but turn yellow at alkaline pH levels (Kruger et al. 1994; Asenstorfer et al. 2006; Fu 2008). Moreover, the presence of protein in the flour is important as it is susceptible to proteolytic activities thus resulting in production of melanin type compounds generated during noodle making detracts the brightness of the product. High protein flour produced Korean noodles that appeared duller because there was less starch available reflects light. The intensity of yellowness and brightness that develops in the alkaline medium is inversely related to the protein content of flours. The protein contents are inversely linked with the brightness of the noodles. The brightness of the noodles tends to decrease with increasing protein contents in wheat flour. It is thus desirable that brighter and YAN should be made from flours of medium protein content. Asenstorfer et al. (2010) examined the darkening in YAN (prepared from different wheat varieties with different levels of polyphenol oxidase (PPO) activity. They were of the view that darkening of noodles is dependent on protein contents and PPO activity that can be reduced using PPO inhibitors, that is, tropolone. However, the rate of darkening of noodles during first few hours was not influenced by protein concentration and PPO activity. After first few hours, the darkening is dependent on protein concentration and PPO activity. Previously, the authors of same research group (Asenstorfer et al. 2009) suggested that the reactive component present in a reasonably high concentration in the soluble protein fraction. Thus tyrosine moieties present in proteins and their oxidation are the main mechanism involved in non-PPO darkening. More recently, the authors has depicted that non-PPO darkening accounted for 69% of total darkening. The PPO enzyme can be inactivated using some solvents and acidic pH. However, PPO cleaves tyrosine at pH of ~8.0 and PPO inhibitors are insensitive to such as tropolone (PPO inhibitors) in the noodle. For the purpose, Australian government is working on project to introduce varieties with and PPO-free and low-PPO activities for their possible utilization in YAN (Asenstorfer et al. 2014). In the case of Japanese raw material, an increase in the level of protein decreases the flour brightness and produces dull noodles. However, this effect is insignificant once the noodle has been cooked, probably because the enzymes are destroyed. The whiteness of Japanese dry noodles also decreased with the increase in protein content. It can be assumed that the tailing starch which contains hemicellulose, phenolics and bran specks and that these components may also explain the fractions functions and their influence on the color tonality of the noodles (Akashi et al. 1999). Although, some artificial colors can also be added to make the product more attractive but these are undesirable entities.

Textural characteristics are also important quality determinants that influence the consumer acceptability of the noodles. Tensile strength also corresponds to elasticity and tenacity for the strain of noodles (Chakraborty et al. 2003), whereas the elasticity modulus refers to the slope of its stress-strain curve. Swelling power is an important index of wheat flour/starch, particularly for its suitability as a small-scale test for predicting noodle eating quality (Crosbie et al. 1999). Although, texture of noodles is a complex character but it can be predicted based on flour quality, water absorption, ingredients used like salt or alkaline reagents as well as processing parameters like sheeting, steaming, and drying method. Many researchers have reported methods and probes for determination of texture for noodles (Hatcher et al. 2009a). Ross and Crosbie (2010) and Ross and Ohm (2006) have reviewed different methods used for textural analysis of noodles and he reported that single test of single machine testing is not suitable to assess the textural profile of the noodles. Several methods and testing devices have been developed for measuring the textural characteristics of cooked noodles. The textural characteristics of cooked noodles can be assessed using Texturometer, Tensiopreser, Instron Universal Testing Machine, and Ottawa Texture Measuring System. Assessment of textural and color profile should match the results from sensory evaluation (Hatcher et al. 2008a; Xue et al. 2010) thus they can be considered as valuable research tools for monitoring noodle texture after changes in formulations, raw materials, and processing. The cutting stress and surface firmness of cooked dry noodles and the breaking stress of uncooked dry noodles are important textural traits to be measured. The internal firmness or cutting stress and surface firmness of cooked noodles showed a significant correlation with sensory firmness of cooked noodles (Bellido and Hatcher 2009). The variations in the texture of the noodles are also dependent on the protein and starch contents of wheat. The microstructure of noodles becomes stiffer with higher amounts of proteins. However, the texture of cooked noodles is more related to the protein network than starch. The internal firmness of cooked noodles and the breaking stress of noodles increased linearly with protein content. The increase in internal firmness of cooked noodles at higher protein levels is due to the tight structure of the noodles which retarded penetration of moisture into the core of noodles during cooking. The tight structure is the result of a strong adhering between the starch and protein components. The gluten fraction is responsible for the change in the cutting characteristics of cooked noodles. Among gluten protein, high-molecular glutenin fraction play more important role. Protein content also plays an important role in determining the cutting and breaking stress of noodles. The surface firmness of cooked dry noodles in contrast is not significantly affected by the protein level. The quality of protein, that is, low molecular weight glutenin fraction is responsible for surface firmness of cooked noodles. Scientists also observed the similar effects of wheat cultivars in Korean dry noodles (Park et al. 2011; Heo et al. 2012).

Eating quality of the boiled noodles is also dependent on starch swelling, for example, surface firmness of YAN is partly influenced by the gelatinization of starch. During the cooking process, the starch granules imbibe water, swell, and gelatinize. The penetration of water and gelatinization of starch depend on the quality of the surrounding protein network. The higher the protein content, the greater the time required for water to penetrate the protein network and gelatinize the starch granules. Likewise, the cooking quality may be defined as the ability to resist disintegration upon prolonged boiling, coupled with a satisfactory degree of cooking and tenderness in the finished product (Shelke et al. 1990). Cooking time is one of the parameters in cooking quality. The optimum cooking time of noodle is defined as the time required for achieving an adequate level of gelatinization which is marked by the disappearance of white center core in a noodle strand. Shelke et al. (1990) stated that noodles with a short cooking time are preferred. The other criterion of cooking quality is cooking loss and it is refers to the amount of solid released from the noodles strands into the cooking water. Cooking caused formation of a weak or discontinuous protein matrix which will allow the leaching of surface materials. Some researchers have studied the cooking loss of noodles (Ugarčić-Hardi et al. 2007). High cooking loss is undesirable as it represents high solubility of starch, resulting in turbid cooking water, low cooking tolerance, and sticky surface and undesirable mouthfeel of final products. Based on these facts, a good cooking quality of noodles and pasta can be defined as the result of high water absorption, low cooking losses with a good texture, that is, high firmness and low stickiness (Bhattacharya and Corke 1996). Morcover, cooking losses are highest in noodles prepared with fine particle size of wheat flour. The losses are also dependent on presence of resistant starches in wheat flour too (Hatcher et al. 2002). Later, Hatcher et al. (2008b) studied the effects of alkaline salts on cooking loss of alkaline noodles. According to them, utilization of sodium hydroxide as alkaline salts is responsible for more than 50% cooking loss as compared to kansui. Moreover, higher amounts of sodium hydroxide also affects the cooking quality. However, utilization of wheat flour with fine particle size could reduce the cooking loss even in the presence of sodium hydroxide (Hatcher et al. 2009a).

The microorganism can influence the quality of the foods along with affecting the health of individuals. The noodles due to their higher moisture contents are more susceptible for microbial spoilage. Although, one or two outbreaks are due to noodles (Tsimogiannis et al. 2001) but still the frequency is far less as compared to fast foods. However, microbiological quality of YAN cannot be ignored. According to the standards mentioned by Garbutt (1997), spoilage appears in food where the growth of bacteria reaches the levels of 10^6 log CFU/g. This is also considered as an important criterion to assess the microbial quality of foods. In this regard, Ghaffar (2009) studied the total aerobic mesophilic bacteria in YAN and reported that on the production day, aerobic mesophilic bacteria ranged from 3 to 4 log CFU/g that increased during subsequent storage and reached up to 6 log CFU/g on the second day of storage at ambient temperature ($28 \pm 2\,^{\circ}$C). Study conducted by Kim et al. (2011) showed that *Bacillus cereus* was the main spoilage bacteria in Korean wet noodles. Similarly, Jensen et al. (2004) found that fresh noodles contained a wide range of spoilage microorganisms including some pathogens such as *Salmonella*, *Staphylococcus aureus*, *E. coli*, and *Listeria monocytogenes*. Moreover, Ghaffar (2009) stated that types of dominating bacteria in YAN produced in Klang Valley, Malaysia, were *Ochrobactrum anthropi*, *Alcaligenes faecalis*, and *Staphylococcus sciuri*.

Chapter 7
Improving the Nutritional Value and Quality

In this heading, efforts are made to highlight the possible measures to improve the nutritional value and quality focusing on the synergistic and antagonistic impact of raw materials and processing techniques. The quality of the product is a result of the combined effect of the raw materials and processing technique. In general, noodles' quality depends largely on flour characteristic, proportion of ingredients, and processing condition used during preparation, or processing variables. So, its understandable for the readers that improving these all factors will lead to improved quality of the products.

The quality determinants of yellow alkaline noodles are mentioned in the previous heading. However, similar parameters are important for enhancing the nutritional values of the noodles too. The yellow alkaline noodles can be prepared with the wheat flour containing appreciable amounts of proteins usually more than 11.0%. For this purpose, the breeding programs are being run by various governments like United States of America (USA), Canada, and Australia. There are several research reports available in these countries focusing on specialized wheat varieties suitable for preparing noodles. In this regard, Ito et al. (2007) evaluated the influence of low PPO wheat Korean cultivar that is, Kitanokaori on yellow alkaline noodle color and physical properties. The cultivar also contains the less amount of amylose. The noodles prepared from its flour showed brightness that didn't reduced to much extent during storage. Moreover, the textural characters showed less breakdown, low setback viscosity, and high elastic indices. Resultantly, the overall acceptability for noodles prepared with Kitanokaori cultivar was also reported higher by the same scientists. As mentioned earlier in the last heading, the darkening of noodles is also dependent on PPO activity, thus governments are working on different project to introduce varieties with, and PPO-free and low-PPO activities for their possible utilization in yellow alkaline noodles. In this regard, some Australian varieties are available in the market with low PPO activities (Asenstorfer et al. 2014).

Utilization of strong flour with high resistance and extensibility in the extensorgraph test can improve the firmness and elasticity of the noodles. The major flour quality requirements that need to be considered in producing bright colored, firm, and elastic noodles are: clean milling, adequate dough strength, protein contents,

© The Authors 2015
R. Karim, M. T. Sultan, *Yellow Alkaline Noodles,* SpringerBriefs in Food,
Health, and Nutrition, DOI 10.1007/978-3-319-12865-8_7

alkaline pH, and optimum starch paste viscosity. Chinese noodles prepared with wheat flour that contain less than 9.5 % protein usually rated poor by the consumer taste panelists. In analyzing the effect of flour characteristics on the quality of Chinese noodles, firmer and more elastic noodles can be produced using flour with higher dough resistance, higher protein content, lower maltose figure, and adequate starch pasting strength. The noodles other than yellow alkaline noodles prepared with protein contents in the range of 9.5 % are more acceptable to the consumers (Park et al. 2011).

Processing aspects of noodle making includes many aspects and many parameters. The textural quality of noodles is dependent mainly on the processing conditions. Surface firmness of cooked noodles increased as roller speeds decreased and reduction percentage increased. The noodles surface was firmer when the dough was pressed between the rollers for a longer time. Dough strength is also related to the chewing and eating quality of noodles. Rapid reduction in dough thickness with few sheeting steps, gives a firmer surface than a more gradual reduction with more sheeting steps. Sheeting of dough causes a rearrangement of the protein network. These rearrangements increased in the number of passages through the rolls. The increased sheeting results in higher water absorption due to higher rate of hydration.

Mixing is one of the most important processing conditions in noodles making process. The increase in mixing time results in breakdown of the surfaces, thus decreasing firmness of noodles. The mixing time is directly linked with the stickiness, as higher the time of mixing, the dough becomes stickier. In the noodles manufacturing, mixing time did not affect the quality of cooked dry noodles. In noodles, the development of gluten is not completed during mixing, but processes of rolling and sheeting are important for complete formation of gluten network. However, main aim of the mixing is to distribute the ingredients and to hydrate the flour particles. Recently, Li et al. (2014) investigated the effects of vacuum mixing on Asian noodle qualities. According to them, the proportion of alkali-soluble proteins increased as compared to decreasing salt-soluble proteins due to vacuum mixing. Moreover, vacuum mixing resulted in more continuous and compact microstructure of gluten proteins in different types of noodles. Resting of dough before sheeting is known to improve dough sheeting properties by allowing uniform moisture distribution and mallowing of wheat gluten (Morris et al. 2000). However, resting is important in noodles where pH is usually less than 7.0. In alkaline noodles, resting period increased surface firmness slightly that remained constant. According to resting of dough before reduction stages, improved the eating quality of Cantonese noodles because it produced smoother and firmer cooked noodles. The improvement in the quality of cooked noodles was due to the presence of more continuous protein matrix in the structure of noodles after compression stages of the rested noodles dough. The combined effect of time and mechanical work in producing constructive and destructive changes on dough properties indicated the importance of controlling processing conditions and variables during noodle making (Ross et al. 1997; Hatcher et al. 2009a).

The cooking quality of noodles and spaghetti is related to the behavior of the product during cooking. The desirable cooking qualities that consumers often look for are the ability to withstand severity of the cooking processes without breaking, minimum disintegration during cooking. Thus, lower cooking losses and sufficient degree of swelling are desirable features for yellow alkaline noodles. Their shape should not be deformed during cooking and noodles should not become too soft on standing after cooking. The amount of solid lost depends on the leaching of surface material, as a result of disruption of the protein matrix at the periphery of the noodles due to vigorous action of the boiling water. Cooking loss, cooked weight, and degree of swelling are significantly correlated to surface stickiness. Although, it is generally believed that poor quality noodles would have greater cooking losses as compared to the good quality noodles (Morris et al. 2000).

The variations in texture of different noodles are dependent on market trends and consumer acceptability. The manufacturer or researchers always focus on consumer's demands, thus traditional values, method of serving, end use quality needs to be focused before designing any improvements. Fewer studies has been conducted to improve the textural characteristics of noodles using modifications of method. In this regard, Thammathongchat et al. (2005) developed a new type of udon noodle that is precooked (gelatinized) only in the center, leaving the surface uncooked (ungelatinized). Such changes would be helpful in quality retention with special reference to texture and firmness. Moreover, Hatcher and Anderson (2007) attempted to optimize the textural profile of yellow alkaline noodles using different alkaline formulation. They observed the parameters like maximum cutting stress (MCS), resistance to compression (RTC), recovery (REC), and stress relaxation time for noodles. According to them, desirable bite (MCS), chewiness (RTC, REC), and relaxation times were achieved with a 1% concentration of alkali salts. According to Moss et al. (1986), addition of alkali salts enhanced the brightness and yellow color tone of the noodles. It is interesting to observe that pH more than 11.0 resulted in better color tonality. However, such alkaline dough holds poor textural profile and tends to break down more rapidly as indicated from the farinograph due to their tougher and stiffer behavior. The recipe can be optimized using 0.3% NaOH or the mixtures of carbonates and thickening agents. Later, Wu et al. (2006) improved the textural characteristics of yellow alkaline noodles as indicated from improved elastic modulus (G') and viscous modulus (G'') using various levels of salt or alkaline (kansui and NaOH) reagents were included in their formulation. The reported that brightest noodles can be obtained with NaOH addition. However, addition of sodium hydroxide results in sticky dough. Therefore, combination of sodium and potassium carbonates are more preferred due to their ability to retain the textural characteristics.

The sensory evaluation of the products is foremost important criteria for determining the quality of the food products. In sensory appraisal, there are many techniques that can be employed for example, consumer acceptability tests, trained taste panel, random marketing testing, etc. As far as the experiments at the institutes are concerned, the use of trained taste panel is more appropriate. Taste panel have been used to evaluate the texture of cooked noodles, pasta, etc. However, the limitations are there in using trained taste panel as genetic variations in individuals are responsible for varying responses. Although, there are various techniques that can be utilized to minimize the variations. The taste panels have been used to evaluate the texture of the cooked noodles and cooked pasta.

The addition or supplementation of natural products is also important to improve the nutritional quality of noodles. However, the proper utilization with better consumer acceptability along with nutrition education is important determinants of success or failure of such nutritional strategies. In this regard, Chang and Wu (2008) prepared fresh Chinese noodles with different levels of green seaweed at 4, 6, and 8%. They were of the view that addition of seaweed enhances the fiber part of noodles thus increasing the water absorption, ultimately leading to higher cooking yields. Moreover, textural properties like breaking energy and capacities of extensibility decreased with the addition of seaweeds. In another study, Ramli et al. (2009) described the utilization of banana pulp and peel flours as functional ingredients in yellow alkaline noodles. The addition of banana decreased the glycaemic index and influenced the physicochemical properties of noodles negatively. However, banana pulp and peel flour further controlled the hydrolysis of starch and enhanced the amounts of dietary fiber in the noodles thus they can be used as functional ingredients for improving the health of the consumers. In a similar study, incorporation of green banana peel and pulp four has been studied by Foo et al. (2011). According to them, addition improved the mechanical and textural properties of the noodles and influenced the breakdown properties of noodles during oral processing. Yeoh et al. (2011) prepared yellow alkaline noodles using cross linkage agents like soy protein isolate, transglutaminase (TG), and ribose. The addition of these ingredients affected the quality of noodles differently for example, lightness increased and yellowish color tonality decreased. However, the products were acceptable (Gan et al. 2009; Bellido and Hatcher 2011). Gulia and Khatkar (2014) prepared noodles from 15 wheat cultivars. According to them, wheat flours containing proteins in the range of 10–12% performed better in noodle making. They also reported that the dough development time and dough stability time are positively correlated with cooking time, hardness, springiness, cohesiveness, and chewiness of noodles overall acceptability. Vijayakumar and Boopathy (2014) prepared the composite flour combinations using whole wheat, tapioca, and defatted soy flour for the noodle preparation. They reported that maximum protein content of 16 g% can be achieved using the combination of 75.54 g of whole wheat flour, 10 g of tapioca flour, and 19.78 g of defatted soy flour. However, the noodles containing higher amounts of soy flour (>10 g) were rated negatively by the consumers. According to them, noodles prepared with composite flour blend containing wheat flour (77.33 g), tapioca (22.19 g), and soy flour (8.92 g) can be used for the preparation of healthy noodles. Gracilaria is seaweed that contains the appreciable amounts of dietary that can be added as ingredient in noodle products. The incorporation of 3% gracilaria seaweed in the noodle ingredients significantly increased their total dietary fiber content (Keyimu 2013). Previously, Ekthamasut (2006) studied the effects of tomato seed meal on the pasting properties of wheat flour and their role in end use quality (alkaline noodle). They observed that tomato seed meal decreased the viscosity and peak time. In addition, the result also revealed that experimental noodles had higher cooking weight, protein, fiber, and lysine content but lower cutting force, L* color and sensory quality than the control. Later, Chin et al. (2012) evaluated that the nutritional quality of yellow alkaline noodles can be improved using surimi powder.

In the nutshell, the quality of noodles can be improved using multilateral approaches for example quality of raw materials, processing conditions, adopting modern techniques, and supplementation with natural products (Fu 2008; Gulia et al. 2014) and condition used during preparation, or processing variables. If all of these variables can be improved than definitely the quality of yellow alkaline noodles can be improved.

Chapter 8
Modern Trends and Innovation

In the recent era, different concepts and developments were made that changed the global scenario of global food market. Several innovations find their application in the processing of food products. These trends include the use of ingredients (natural products, herbal noodles, functional noodles, antioxidants, and antimicrobial agents), processing equipments, and conditions (nonthermal processing, microwave, ultrasonic, irradiation, parboiling, etc.). Similarly, the scientific advancements helped the noodles industry to overcome some problems. Moreover, the consumer convenience and marketing tactics also changed with the passage of time. Now, the consumers are more concerned with their health and concepts of food safety. However, the research studies are still required to commercialize the research findings in comprehendible manner.

Yellow alkaline noodles contain high moisture contents thus have lower shelf life and are more prone to microbial spoilage. Under normal conditions, the shelf life of the noodles is around 1–1.5 days. The spoilage can result in off color, odor, and slime production. Spoilage is always related to the growth of bacteria, followed by yeast, and moulds. Besides containing high moisture content, pH of yellow alkaline noodles is more than 9.0 that also cause the growth of the moulds. Shorter shelf life of such noodles is also causing problems for the industries as there are two possible threats that is, waste and chances of food poisoning. In other products, the chemical preservatives are added but there are several issues nowadays that demands products free from chemical preservatives. Although, natural antioxidants/antimicrobial agents may enhance the shelf life of the noodles, but still it lacks any significance for large-scale industries.

The concepts of food spoilage are not newer, as people of old civilizations were also aware about them. They were also using some traditional methods to control the spoilage. In the last two centuries, the food preservation gained immense success. However, the side effects associated with some preservation techniques resulted in mass investigations to design some modern techniques or optimize some old practices, thus a balance could be achieved that is, retention of nutritional value and enhancing the shelf life of the products (Rahman 2007). However, some concepts

R. Karim, M. T. Sultan, *Yellow Alkaline Noodles,* SpringerBriefs in Food, Health, and Nutrition, DOI 10.1007/978-3-319-12865-8_8

need to be understood and among them is the mode of spoilage that is physical, chemical, and microbiological. These all means require different techniques. According to Devlieghere et al. (2004), food preservation is a continuous fight to protect the foods from spoilage agents. The techniques which are currently employed globally include salting, heat transfer, pH modification, and modifying the environments using some chemicals. However, all of them have some advantages and disadvantages (Takashima et al. 2006).

Hurdle technology is a newer concept in the domain of food processing and preservation. In this method, different hurdles (preservation techniques) are applied to reduce the spoilage and deteriorative changes occurring in the food products. These techniques include use of acidic pH, ingredients variations, natural antioxidants, and antimicrobial agents. Moreover, the modern tools like microwave, UV treatment, ozone gas sterilization, ultrasonic, and irradiation can be utilized to enhance the shelf life of the yellow alkaline noodles (Devlieghere et al. 2004; Takashima et al. 2006; Xue et al. 2008). As far as yellow alkaline noodles are concerned, they have shelf life of few hours to few days thus preservation techniques should be selected accordingly. The treatments like γ-irradiation, microwave, and pulsed-UV treatment have the potential to be applied as the postprocessing decontamination. Li et al. (2013) studies the effects of ozone treatment on the presence of microorganism in wheat flour and shelf life of fresh noodles. They were of the view that total plate count (TPC) can be largely reduced in wheat flour exposed to ozone gas for 30 and 60 min along with increasing the wheat whiteness. Moreover, dough stability and peak viscosity of wheat starch were all increased by ozone treatment. Additionally, ozone treated noodles were generally higher in firmness, springiness, and chewiness, while lower in adhesiveness. The growths of microorganism and enzymes activities were also decreased as a function of ozone treatment. Xu et al. (2010) explored the role of flaxseed as a food preservative against the fungal strains of *Penicillium chrysogenum, Aspergillus flavus, Fusarium graminearum*, and a *Penicillium sp.* isolated from molded noodles. They reported that flaxseed at 9 % or higher concentrations reduced the mold count of fresh noodle during storage. It can be claimed that flaxseed holding antimicrobial activity can be used as functional ingredient to render multiple benefits. Later, Li et al. (2011) studied the effect of water activity (aw), irradiation, and their combinations. They observed that the TPC (total plate count) never exceeded the selected deterioration threshold limit (10^6 CFU/g) at irradiation dose of 4 kGy or higher. Moreover, noodles irradiated at 4 kGy showed the best pH and sensory stability. In chemical treatment, combination of glycerol (3 %), propylene glycol (2 %), compound phosphate (0.4 %), and salt (3 %) was highly effective in reducing the aw. It can be concluded that the antimicrobial effect of preservation can be optimized by combining several techniques (hurdle technology). Application of hurdle technology allows the usage of lower energy level thus maintaining the food quality.

In the last heading, it has been discussed already that various scientists attempted to enhance the nutritional values of alkaline noodles using various products, that is, green seaweed (Chang and Wu 2008), banana peel and pulp (Ramli et al. 2009), soy protein isolate (Yeoh et al. 2011), and tapioca and defatted soy flour (Vijayakumar and Boopathy 2014). In all these studies, focus was to increase the nutritional values of the noodles with special reference to antioxidants, dietary fiber, and high quality proteins. The use of nutraceutical and functional components are also gaining wide range of acceptance among the masses. In this regard, various scientists made the efforts to incorporate soy proteins, dietary fiber, sweet potato flour, etc., to enhance the nutritional value of the yellow alkaline noodles.

Conclusion

The production of high quality noodles and pasta products have been associated largely with particular physicochemical properties of the protein components in the dough. Other flour constituents and added ingredients also influence the desirable characteristics and organoleptic qualities. The optimized conditions of constituents, ingredients, and processing techniques would give the optimum quality of yellow alkaline noodles.

© The Authors 2015
R. Karim, M. T. Sultan, *Yellow Alkaline Noodles,* SpringerBriefs in Food, Health, and Nutrition, DOI 10.1007/978-3-319-12865-8

References

Ahmad I, Anjum FM, Butt MS, Bajwa BE (2007) Improvement in spring wheat quality in Pakistan. Pakistan J Agric Res 20(1/2):1–6

Akashi H, Takahashi M, Endo S (1999) Evaluation of starch properties of wheats used for Chinese yellow-alkaline noodles in Japan. Cereal Chem 76(1):50–55

Arif S, Ahmed M, Khanzada KK (2006) Quality evaluation of some sindh (Pakistan) wheat varieties. II. Correlation among various quality traits. Pak J Sci Ind Res 49(4):285–289

Asenstorfer RE, Wang Y, Mares DJ (2006) Chemical structure of flavonoid compounds in wheat (*Triticum aestivum* L.) flour that contribute to the yellow colour of Asian alkaline noodles. J Cereal Sci 43(1):108–119

Asenstorfer RE, Appelbee MJ, Mares DJ (2009) Physical–Chemical analysis of non-polyphenol oxidase (Non-PPO) darkening in yellow alkaline noodles. J Agric Food Chem 57(12):5556–5562

Asenstorfer RE, Appelbee MJ, Mares DJ (2010) Impact of protein on darkening in yellow alkaline noodles. J Agric Food Chem 58:4500–4507

Asenstorfer RE, Appelbee MJ, Kusznir CA, Mares DJ (2014) Towards an understanding of mechanisms involved non-PPO darkening in yellow alkaline noodles (YAN). J Agric Food Chem 62:4725–4730

Baik BK, Lee MR (2003) Effect of starch amylose content of wheat on textural properties of white salted noodles. Cereal Chem 80:304–9

Bellido GG, Hatcher DW (2009) Stress relaxation behaviour of yellow alkaline noodles: effect of deformation history. J food Eng 93(4):460–467

Bellido GG, Hatcher DW (2011) Effects of a cross-linking enzyme on the protein composition, mechanical properties, and microstructure of Chinese-style noodles. Food chem 125(3):813–822

Bhattacharya M, Corke H (1996) Selection of desirable starch pasting properties in wheat for use in white salted or yellow alkaline noodles. Cereal Chem 73(6):721–728

Chakraborty M, Hareland GA, Manthey FA, Berglund LR (2003) Evaluating quality of yellow alkaline noodles made from mechanically abraded sprouted wheat. J Sci Food Agric 83(5):487–495

Chang HC, Wu LC (2008) Texture and quality properties of Chinese fresh egg noodles formulated with green seaweed (*Monostroma nitidum*) powder. J Food Sci 73(8):S398–S404

Chin CK, Huda N, Yang TA (2012) Incorporation of surimi powder in wet yellow noodles and its effects on the physicochemical and sensory properties. Int Food Res J 2:701–707

Chung CE, Lee KW, Cho MS (2010) Noodle consumption patterns of American consumers: NHANES 2001–2002. Nutr Res Pract 4(3):243–251

Cole ME (1991) Prediction and measurement of pasta quality. Int J Food Sci Technol 26(2):133–151

© The Authors 2015

R. Karim, M. T. Sultan, *Yellow Alkaline Noodles,* SpringerBriefs in Food, Health, and Nutrition, DOI 10.1007/978-3-319-12865-8

Crosbie GB, Ross AS, Moro T, Chiu PC (1999) Starch and protein quality requirements of Japanese alkaline noodles (Ramen). Cereal Chem 76(3):328–334

Deng Z, Tian J, Zhao L, Zhang Y, Sun C (2008) High temperature-induced changes in high molecular weight glutenin subunits of Chinese winter wheat and its influences on the texture of Chinese noodles. J Agron Crop Sci 194(4):262–269

Devlieghere F, Vermeiren L., Debevere J (2004) New preservation technologies: possibility and limitation. Int Dairy J 14:273–285

Edwards NM, Scanlon MG, Kruger JE, Dexter JE (1996) Oriental noodle dough rheology: relationship to water absorption, formulation, and work input during dough sheeting. Cereal Chem 73:708–711

Ekthamasut K (2006) Effect of tomato seed meal on wheat pasting properties and alkaline noodle qualities. Aust J Technol 9:147–152

Foo WT, Yew HS, Liong MT, Azhar ME (2011) Influence of formulations on textural, mechanical and structural breakdown properties of cooked yellow alkaline noodles. Int Food Res J 18(4):1295–1301

Fu BX (2008) Asian noodles: history, classification, raw materials, and processing. Food Res Int 41(9):888–902

Fuerst EP, Anderson JV, Morris CF (2006) Delineating the role of polyphenol oxidase in the darkening of alkaline wheat noodles. J Agric Food Chem 54(6):2378–2384

Galvez FCF, Resurreccion AV (1992) Reliability of the focus group technique in determining the quality characteristics of mungbean [*Vigna radiata* (L.) wilczec] noodles. J Sens Stud 7(4):315–326

Gan CY, Ong WH, Wong LM, Easa AM (2009) Effects of ribose, microbial transglutaminase and soy protein isolate on physical properties and in-vitro starch digestibility of yellow noodles. LWT-Food Sci Technol 42(1):174–179

Garbutt J (1997) Essentials of food microbiology. Hodder Headline Group, London, pp 124–129

Ghaffar S, Abdulamir AS, Bakar FA, Karim R, Saari N (2009) Microbial growth, sensory characteristic and pH as potential spoilage indicators of Chinese yellow wet noodles from commercial processing plants. Am J Appl Sci 6(6):1059

Gulia N, Khatkar BS (2014) Relationship of dough thermomechanical properties with oil uptake, cooking and textural properties of instant fried noodles. Food Sci Technol Int 20(3):171–182

Gulia N, Dhaka V, Khatkar BS (2014) Instant noodles: processing, quality, and nutritional aspects. Crit Rev Food Sci Nutr 54(10):1386–1399

Hatcher DW, Anderson MJ (2007) Influence of alkaline formulation on oriental noodle color and texture 1. Cereal Chem 84(3):253–259

Hatcher DW, Kruger JE, Anderson MJ (1999) Influence of water absorption on the processing and quality of oriental noodles. Cereal Chem 76:566–572

Hatcher DW, Anderson MJ, Desjardins RG, Edwards NM, Dexter JE (2002) Effects of flour particle size and starch damage on processing and quality of white salted noodles. Cereal Chem 79(1):64–71

Hatcher DW, Bellido GG, Dexter JE, Anderson MJ, Fu BX (2008a) Investigation of uniaxial stress relaxation parameters to characterize the texture of yellow alkaline noodles made from durum and common wheats. J Texture Stud 39:695–708

Hatcher DW, Edwards NM, Dexter JE (2008b) Effects of particle size and starch damage of flour and alkaline reagent on yellow alkaline noodle characteristics. Cereal chem 85(3):425–432

Hatcher DW, Dexter JE, Anderson MJ, Bellido GG, Fu BX (2009a) Effect of blending durum wheat flour with hard white wheat flour on the quality of yellow alkaline noodles. Food Chem 113(4):980–988

Hatcher DW, Bellido GG, Anderson MJ (2009b) Flour particle size, starch damage, and alkali reagent: impact on uniaxial stress relaxation parameters of yellow alkaline noodles. Cereal Chem 86(3):361–368

Heo H, Kang CS, Woo SH, Lee KS, Choo BK, Park CS (2012) Characteristics of yellow alkaline noodles prepared from Korean wheat cultivar. Food Sci Biotechnol 21(1):69–81

Hou G (2001) Oriental noodles. Adv Food Nutr Res 43:141–193

Hou GG (2010) Asian noodles: science, technology, and processing. Wiley

Hou G, Kruk M (1998) Asian noodle technology. Tech Bull 20(12):1–10

Huang YC, Lai HM (2010) Noodle quality affected by different cereal starches. J Food Eng 97(2):135–143

Huang S, Morrison WR (1988) Aspects of proteins in Chinese and British common (hexaploid) wheats related to quality of white and yellow Chinese noodles. J Cereal Sci 8(2):177–187

Hung PV, Hatcher DW (2011) Ultra-performance liquid chromatography (UPLC) quantification of carotenoids in durum wheat: influence of genotype and environment in relation to the colour of yellow alkaline noodles (YAN). Food Chem 125(4):1510–1516

Ito M, Ohta K, Nishio Z, Tabiki T, Hashimoto N, Funatsuki W, Miura H, Yamauchi H (2007) Quality evaluation of yellow alkaline noodles made from the Kitanokaori wheat cultivar. Food Sci Technol Res 13(3):253–260

Jensen N, Hocking AD, Miskelly D, Berghofer LK (2004) Microbiological safety of high moisture noodles. 1. Marketplace survey of noodles sold in Australia. Food Aust 56(3):71–74

Jiang H, Martin J, Okot-Kotber M, Seib PA (2011) Color of whole-wheat foods prepared from a bright-white hard winter wheat and the phenolic acids in its coarse bran. J Food Sci 76(6):C846–C852

Jun WJ, Seib PA, Chung OK (1998) Characteristics of noodle flours from Japan. Cereal Chem 75:820–825

Keyimu XG (2013) The effects of using seaweed on the quality of Asian noodles. J Food Process Technol 4(216):2

Kim BY, Lee JY, Ha SD (2011) Growth characteristics and development of a predictive model for *Bacillus cereus* in fresh wet noodles with added ethanol and thiamine. J Food Prot® 74(4):658–664

Konik CM, Mikkelsen LM, Moss R, Gore PJ (1994) Relationship between physical starch properties and yellow alkaline noodle quality. Starch 46:292–299

Kruger JE, Matsuo RR, Preston K (1992) A comparison of methods for the prediction of Cantonese noodle colour. Can J Plant Sci 72:1021–1029

Kruger JE, Hatcher DW, DePauw R (1994) A whole seed assay for polyphenol oxidase in Canadian prairie spring wheats and its usefulness as a measure of noodle darkening. Cereal Chem 71(4):324–326

Li M, Zhu K, Guo X, Peng W, Zhou H (2011) Effect of water activity (aw) and irradiation on the shelf-life of fresh noodles. Innov Food Sci Emerg Technol 12(4):526–530

Li M, Peng J, Zhu KX, Guo XN, Zhang M, Peng W, Zhou HM (2013) Delineating the microbial and physical-chemical changes during storage of ozone treated wheat flour. Innovative Food Sci Emerg Technol 20:223–229

Li M, Zhu KX Peng J, Guo XN, Amza T, Peng W, Zhou HM (2014) Delineating the protein changes in Asian noodles induced by vacuum mixing. Food Chem 143:9–16

McCormick KM, Panozzo JF, Hong SH (1991) A swelling power test for selecting potential noodle quality wheats. Crop Pasture Sci 42(3):317–323

Miskelly DM, Moss HJ (1985) Flour quality requirements for chinese noodle manufacture. J Cereal Sci 3(4):379–387

Morris CF, Jeffers HC, Engle DA (2000) Effect of processing, formula and measurement variables on alkaline noodle color-toward an optimized laboratory system. Cereal Chem 77(1):77–85

Moss HJ, Miskelly DM, Moss R (1986) The effect of alkaline conditions on the properties of wheat flour dough and Cantonese-style noodles. J Cereal Sci 4(3):261–268

Okusu H, Otsubo S, Dexter J, Hou GG (2010) Wheat milling and flour quality analysis for noodles in Japan. In: Hou GG (ed) Asian noodles: science, technology, and processing. Wiley, New Jersey, pp 57–73

Ong YL, Ross AS, Engle DA (2010) Glutenin macropolymer in salted and alkaline noodle doughs. Cereal Chemistry 87(1):79–85

Park CS, Baik BK (2004) Relationship between protein characteristics and instant noodle making quality of wheat flour. Cereal Chem 81:159–164

Park CS, Hong BH, Baik BK (2003) Protein quality of wheat desirable for making fresh white salted noodles and its influences on processing and texture of noodles. Cereal Chem 80(3):297–303

Park CS, Kang CS, Jeung JU, Woo SH (2011) Influence of allelic variations in glutenin on the quality of pan bread and white salted noodles made from Korean wheat cultivars. Euphytica 180(2):235–250

Rahman MS (2007) Handbook of food preservation, 2nd edn. CRC Press, Boca Raton

Ramli S, Alkarkhi AF, Shin Yong Y, Min-Tze L, Easa AM (2009) Effect of banana pulp and peel flour on physicochemical properties and in vitro starch digestibility of yellow alkaline noodles. Int J Food Sci Nutr 60(s4):326–340

Rayas-Duarte P, Francisco C, Payton ME, Bellmer DD, Carver BF, Huang WN (2009) Alkaline noodles and flour/gel properties of hard red and white winter wheat. J Food Qual 32(5):627–643

Ross AS, Crosbie GB (2010) Effects of flour characteristics on noodle texture. In: Hou GG (ed) Asian noodles: science, technology, and processing. Wiley, New Jersey, pp 313–330

Ross AS, Ohm JB (2006) Sheeting characteristics of salted and alkaline Asian noodle doughs: comparison with lubricated squeezing flow attributes. Cereal Foods World 51:191–196

Ross AS, Quail KJ, Crosbie GB (1997) Physicochemical properties of Australian flours influencing the texture of yellow alkaline noodles. Cereal Chem 78:814–820

Rosyid TA, Karim R, Adzahan NM, Ghazali FM (2011) Antibacterial activity of several Malaysian leaves extracts on the spoilage bacteria of yellow alkaline noodles. Afr J Microbiol Res 5:898–904

Shelke K, Dick JW, Holm YR, Loo KS (1990) Chinese wet noodle formulation: a response surface methodology study. Cereal Chem 67(4):338–342

Shewry PR (2009) Wheat. J Exp Bot 60(6):1537–53

Takashima H, Miyakawa Y, Kanno Y (2007) Microwave sterilization with metal thin film coated catalyst in liquid phase. Mater Sci Eng C 27(4):898–903

Thammathongchat S, Fukuoka M, Watanabe H (2005) An innovative noodle: gelatinized at the core, leaving the surface ungelatinized. J Food Eng 70(1):27–33

Toyokawa H, Rubenthaler GL, Powers JR, Schanus EG (1989a) Japanese noodle qualities. I. Flour component. Cereal Chem 66:382–386

Toyokawa H, Rubenthaler GL, Powers J. R, Schanus EG (1989b) Japanese noodle qualities. II. Starch component. Cereal Chem 66:387–391

Tsimogiannis H, Mmolawa P, Davos D, Tribe IG (2001) An outbreak of *Salmonella typhimurium* phage type 29 linked to a noodle restaurant in South Australia. Commun Dis Intell Q Report 25(2):72–76

Ugarcic-Hardi Z, Jukic M, Komlenic DK, Sabo M, Hardi J (2007) Quality parameters of noodles made with various supplements. Czech J Food Sci 25:151–157

Veraverbeke WS, Delcour JA (2002) Wheat protein composition and properties of wheat glutenin in relation to breadmaking functionality. Crit Rev Food Sci Nutr 42(3):179–208

Vijayakumar TP, Boopathy P (2012) Optimization of ingredients for noodle preparation using response surface methodology. J Food Sci Technol 51(8):1501–1508

Wang YH, Lu XT, Wang JW (2008) Relationship between the wheat-powder descent amount and the damaged starch content and the bud rate. J Chang Chun Univ Technol (Natural Science Edition) 29:455–458

World Instant Noodle Association Expanding Market (2013) World instant noodle association. Osaka, Japan. http://instantnoodles.org/noodles/expanding-market.html

Wu J, Beta T, Corke H (2006) Effects of salt and alkaline reagents on dynamic rheological properties of raw oriental wheat noodles. Cereal Chem 83(2):211–217

Xu Y, Hall C III, Wolf-Hall C, Manthey F (2008) Fungistatic activity of flaxseed in potato dextrose agar and a fresh noodle system. Int J Food Microbiol 121(3):262–267

Xue C, Sakai N, Fukuoka M. (2008) Use of microwave heating to control the degree of starch gelatinization in noodles. J Food Eng 87(3):357–362

Xue DAN, Gao H, Zhao LEI, Yin J (2010) Relationships between instrumental measurements and sensory evaluation in instant noodles studied by partial least squares regression. J Texture Stud 41(2):224–241

Yamauchi H, Ito M, Nishio Z, Tabiki T, Kim SJ, Hashimoto N, Hideho Miura H, ISM Z (2007) Effects of high-molecular-weight glutenin subunits on the texture of yellow alkaline noodles using near-isogenic lines. Food Sci Technol Res 13(3):227–234

Ye Y, Zhang Y, Yan J, Zhang Y, He Z, Huang S, Quail KJ (2009) Effects of flour extraction rate, added water, and salt on color and texture of Chinese white noodles. Cereal Chem 86(4):477–485

Yeoh SY, Alkarkhi AF, Ramli SB, Easa AM (2011) Effect of cooking on physical and sensory properties of fresh yellow alkaline noodles prepared by partial substitution of wheat flour with soy protein isolate and treated with cross-linking agents. Int J Food Sci Nutr 62(04):410–417

Zeb A, Zahir A, Ahmad T, Abdumanon A (2006) Physiochemical characteristics of wheat varieties growing in the same and different ecological regions of Pakistan. Pakistan J Agric Biol Sci 9(9):1823–1828

Zhang SB, Lu QY, Yang H, Meng DD (2011) Effects of protein content, glutenin-to-gliadin ratio, amylose content, and starch damage on textural properties of Chinese fresh white noodles. Cereal Chem 88(3):296–301

Zhao LF, Seib PA (2005) Alkaline-carbonate noodles from hard winter wheat flours varying in protein, swelling power, and polyphenol oxidase activity. Cereal Chem 82(5):504–516